2019 GLUTEN FREE BUYERS GUIDE

JOSH SCHIEFFER

Table of Contents

Introduction by Josh Schieffer

First, let me thank you for picking up this book. We are delighted you have decided to find the best in gluten-free. This book has been carefully designed to help you quickly connect with the best gluten-free products, people, services, and organizations. We host the Annual Gluten-Free Awards; a program that enables the gluten-free community to cast votes for their favorites. This year we had 8,971 people take part in the voting process. The 272,471 individual responses are all rolled up in the following pages.

This year we changed the cover design and added a few new award categories now totaling 58.

HOW THE GLUTEN FREE AWARDS WORK

Presented by The Gluten Free Buyers Guide

PRODUCT REGISTRATION

Gluten Free Buyers Guide Registration

Each year brands register their products in The Gluten Free Buyers Guide. The guide consists of 60 gluten free categories ranging from gluten free bread to gluten free comfort food. Find more registration details at GlutenFreeBuyersGuide.com

GLUTEN FREE BLOGGERS & INFLUENCERS

Top bloggers & influences register products

We generate a list of 20-30 top gluten free bloggers and social media influencers. We ask them to register their favorite brands and products to be submitted into The Gluten Free Buyers Guide.

COMMUNITY VOTE

We ask the gluten free community to vote

Once we have the products registered for The Gluten Free Buyers Guide we create a voting ballot with those products listed in their respected categories. Nearly 10,000 people in the gluten free community vote for their favorites.

PUBLISHING

We publish The Gluten Free Buyers Guide

The Gluten Free Buyers Guide publishes all products that had been registered highlighting the top three GFA Award Winners in each category. The winners will have an image of their product so consumers can quickly identify those products while shopping.

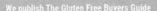

LEARN MORE AT GLUTENFREEBUYERSGUIDE.COM
OR
THEGLUTENFREEAWARDS.COM

2

Our Story

The story behind The Gluten Free Awards that very few people know

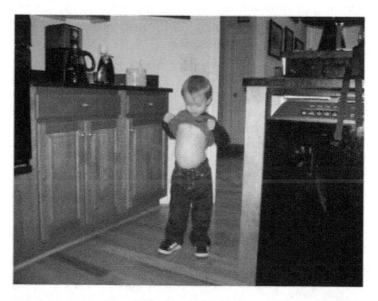

I remember it like it was yesterday when my four-year-old son Jacob, now thirteen, was playing in the kiddie pool with other kids that I assumed were his age based on their height. After asking all the surrounding kids what ages they were, I realized Jacob was significantly smaller than kids his own age. This prompted my wife and I to seek a professional opinion. After consulting with our family physician, she confirmed that Jacob had essentially stopped growing for an entire year without us realizing it. He was referred to Jeff Gordon's Children's Hospital in Charlotte North Carolina to discuss possible growth hormone therapy. The doctors there reviewed Jacob's case and requested a few blood tests based on some suspicions they had.

Our cell phone service at our house was terrible so when the doctor finally called with the blood results, my wife and I ran to the front of the driveway to hear the doctor clearly. With a sporadic signal, we heard "Jacob has celiac disease." We looked at each other as tears ran down my wife's face. We huddled closer to the phone and asked, "what is celiac disease?". After getting a brief description mixed with crappy cell service and happy neighbors waving as they drove by, my wife and I embraced and wept. We were told to maintain his normal diet until we could have an endoscopy and biopsy for further confirmation. Once confirmed our next visit was to a registered dietitian for guidance.

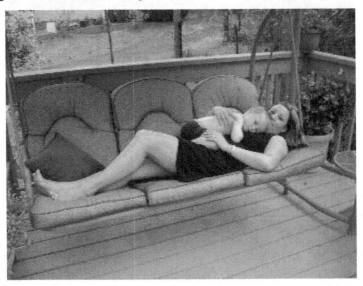

Jayme, my wife, made the appointment and called me with a weird request. "Will you meet me at the dietitian's house for a consultation?". I was confused when she said to go to her house. Jayme then explained that the dietician's daughter had celiac disease too and the best way to show the new lifestyle to patients would be to dive right in. I'll admit, it was a bit uncomfortable at first to be in a strangers' house looking at their personal items but looking back now, I wouldn't change it for the world. That encounter is ultimately the motivation behind The Gluten Free Awards and the associated Gluten Free Buyers Guide. We left her house with complete understanding of cross contamination, best practices and what products they personally liked and disliked. That visit was life changing and left us feeling confident as we made our way to the local health food store.

That first trip shopping took forever. Each label was read, and cross checked with our list of known gluten containing suspects. It was also shocking to see the bill when it was time to pay. We had replaced our entire pantry and fridge with all products that had the "Gluten Free" label. We both worked full-time and had decent paying jobs and it still set us back financially.

We looked for support groups locally and came across a "100% Gluten-Free Picnic" in Raleigh, which was two hours away from where we lived. This was our first time meeting other people with celiac disease and we were fortunate to have met some informative people that were willing to help with the hundreds of questions we had. We were introduced to a family whose son had been recently diagnosed with celiac disease as well. His condition was much worse than Jacobs and he was almost hospitalized before finally being diagnosed. They confided in us as we shared similar stories. There were two differences that would change my life forever. The first was the fact that they didn't have the same experience with a registered dietitian. Instead they were handed a two-page Xerox copy of "safe foods". Second, they didn't have the financial security to experiment with gluten free counterparts. Their first two months exposed to the gluten free life style left them extremely depressed and broke.

On our way home from that picnic, Jayme and I felt compelled to help make a difference in some way. We were determined to help that family and others being diagnosed with this disease. Up until that day, we hadn't found a resource that gave unbiased opinions on gluten free products and services. Fast forward a few years and I too was diagnosed with celiac disease. That year, The Gluten Free Awards were born.

Originally our vision was to create a one-page website with a handful of categories organized by peoples' favorites. Since 2010 we have produced The Annual Gluten Free Awards (GFA) growing into sixty gluten free categories. After several requests, in 2014, we took the GFA results and published our first Gluten Free Buyers Guide. The annual guide is sold primarily in the United States however we continue to see increased global sales. Each year we have over 3,000 people vote for their favorite gluten free products and we now communicate to nearly 20,000 people weekly through our email list and social media channels.

We want to thank those special people and organizations that brought us to where we are today:

Pat Fogarty MS, RD, LDN for allowing us to enter your home.

Jeff Gordon's Children's Hospital

Raleigh Celiac Support Groups

Rebecca Panuski, MD

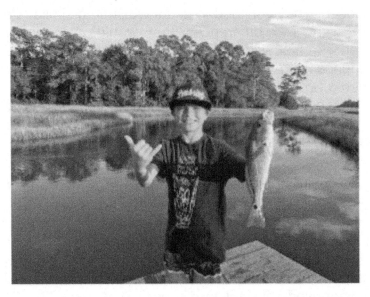

I hope you have learned something new from the story behind The Gluten Free Awards. Today, Jacob and I continue to live a healthy gluten free lifestyle.

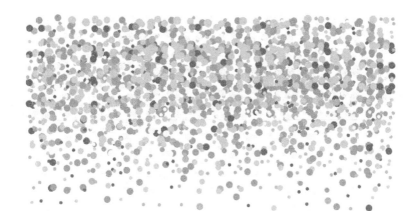

Celebrating 10 Years of connecting the gluten free community to the best products, people and services. THANK YOU!

Best Gluten Free Bagels

9th Annual Gluten-Free Awards:

1st Place Winner: Canyon Bakehouse Everything Bagels

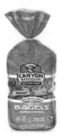

2nd Place Winner: ALDI: liveGfree Gluten Free Bagels - Cinnamon Raisin

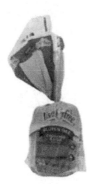

3rd Place Winner: ALDI: liveGfree Gluten Free Bagels - Plain

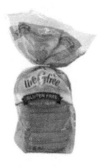

Other Great Products:

Promise - Gluten-Free Plain Bagels

The Greater Knead - Plain Gluten Free Bagel

Wheat's End New York Style Bagels

Ducks and Dragons Flourless Poppy Seed Bagel

Best Gluten Free Beer Brands

9th Annual Gluten-Free Awards:

1st Place Winner: Redbridge

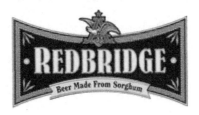

2nd Place Winner: Glutenberg

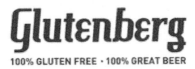

3rd Place Winner: Ghostfish Brewing Company

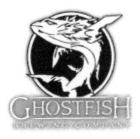

Other Great Products:

Green's

Bards

Ground Breaker Brewing

Best Gluten Free Bloggers & Influencers

9th Annual Gluten-Free Awards:

1st Place Winner: Jules Shepard https://gfjules.com/

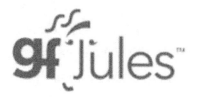

2nd   Place   Winner: Nicole   Hunn
https://glutenfreeonashoestring.com/

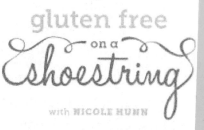

3rd Place Winner: Gluten Dude https://gluten͏   ͏com/

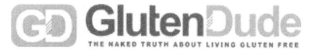

Other Great Bloggers and Influencers:

Erica Dermer http://www.celiacandthebeast.com/

Tricia Thompson, MS, RD
https://www.glutenfreewatchdog.org/

Elana Amsterdam http://www.elanaspantry.com/

Anti-Wheat girl http://antiwheatgirl.com/

Erin Smith https://glutenfreeglobetrotter.com
and https://glutenfreefun.blogspot.com/

Jackie Aanonsen McEwan
https://www.glutenfreefollowme.com/

Diana Duangnet http://www.travelfarglutenfree.com/

Rachael Hunt http://www.glutenfreedominc.com/

Taylor Miller https://www.halelifeblog.com/

Melinda Arcara http://www.glutenfreebebe.com/

Shay Lachendro https://www.whattheforkfoodblog.com/

Pam Jordan http://www.imaceliac.com/

Michael Frolichstein http://www.celiacproject.com/

Nicole Cogan https://nobread.com/

Lori Miller https://glutenfreeglobalicious.com/

Jessica Hanson https://tastymeditation.wordpress.com/

Esther Trevino https://theglutenfreenerd.com/

Rebecca Pytell https://strengthandsunshine.com/

Christina Kantzavelos https://www.buenqamino.com/

Jackie Ourman http://jackieourman.com/

Sema Dibooglu http://eatwithoutgluten.blogspot.com/

Aly Mang http://thebalancedbeauty.com/

Best Gluten Free Books

9th Annual Gluten-Free Awards:

1st Place Winner: The First Year: Celiac Disease and Living Gluten-Free: An Essential Guide for the Newly Diagnosed: Jules Shepard

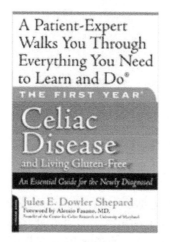

2nd Place Winner: Gluten Is My Bitch: Rants, Recipes, and Ridiculousness for the Gluten-Free by April Peveteaux

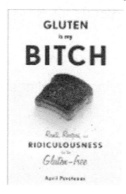

3rd Place Winner: Jennifer's Way: My Journey with Celiac Disease--What Doctors Don't Tell You and How You Can Learn to Live Again by Jennifer Esposito

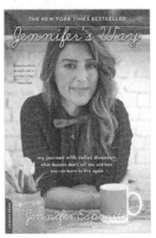

Other Great Books:

Gluten Freedom: The Nation's Leading Expert Offers the Essential Guide to a Healthy, Gluten-Free Lifestyle by Alessio Fasano (Author), Susie Flaherty (Contributor)

Celiac and the Beast: A Love Story Between a Gluten-Free Girl, Her Genes, and a Broken Digestive Tract by Erica Dermer

Dough Nation by Nadine Grzeskowiak

3 Steps to Gluten-Free Living by Melinda Arcara

Best Gluten Free Bread Brands

9th Annual Gluten-Free Awards:

1st Place Winner: Canyon Bakehouse 7-Grain Bread

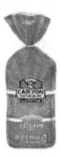

2nd Place Winner: Trader Joe's Gluten Free White Bread

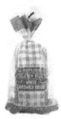

3rd Place Winner: Canyon Bakehouse Gluten Free Hawaiian Sweet Bread

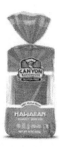

Other Great Products:

ALDI: liveGfree Gluten Free Bread - White

ALDI: liveGfree Gluten Free Bread - Whole Grain

Three Bakers' 7 Ancient Grains

BFree Soft White Sandwich Loaf

Three Bakers' White Bread

Three Bakers' Great Seed

Promise Gluten Free Rosemary & Olive Oil Sourdough Loaf

Promise Gluten Free Rustic White Sourdough Loaf

Food For Life Gluten Free Rice Pecan Bread

Promise Gluten Free 7 Seeds Sourdough Loaf

Lidl Gluten Free Cinnamon Raisin Bread

Lidl Gluten Free White Bread

Promise Gluten Free Seeds and Fruit Sourdough Loaf

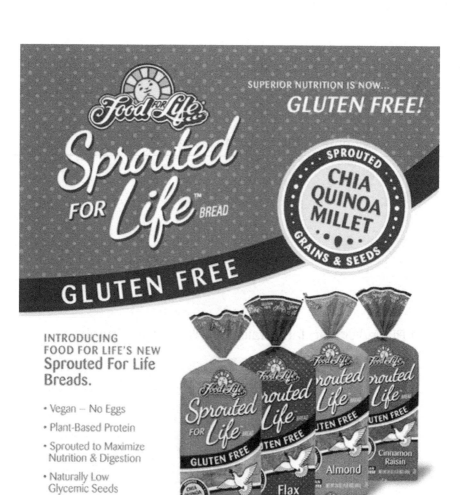
17

Best Gluten Free Bread Crumbs

9th Annual Gluten-Free Awards:

1st Place Winner: Glutino Bread Crumbs

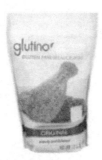

2nd Place Winner: Ian's Italian Panko Bread Crumbs

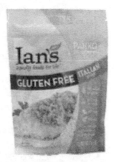

3rd Place Winner: Schar Gluten Free Bread Crumbs

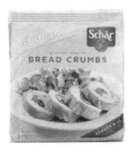

Other Great Products:

Aleia's Gluten Free Foods Bread Crumbs

Katz Gluten Free Bread Crumbs

Gillian's Foods Gluten Free Italian Bread Crumbs

DID YOU KNOW?

30-50% OF WORLD POPULATION HAS GENETIC PREDISPOSITION TO CELIAC DISEASE

Quoted from:
17th International Celiac Disease
Symposium in New Delhi, India

Spinach Artichoke Dip

Pam Jordan, creator of I'm A Celiac (imaceliac.com)

Grab some tasty Gluten Free crackers and dig into this baked Spinach Artichoke dip that has all the components you remember.

I created this recipe for a "Date Night In" with the Hubby. With 3 kiddos, date nights out can get pricey and take a lot of coordination with sitters. We have found that making a tasty meal at home once the kiddos are in bed is a great way to have a date and save money.

For our date I made this Spinach Artichoke dip, steak, roasted veggies and finished it off with carrot cake. It was a big hit!

Spinach Artichoke Dip

Ingredients

8 oz cream cheese, softened

1 cup artichoke hearts, chopped

2 cups frozen spinach, thawed and drained

1/2 cup shredded parmesan cheese

1/2 cup shredded mozzarella cheese

1 tsp GF bouillon

Salt and pepper

1/2 GF bread crumbs

Instructions

Heat oven to 350 degrees.

In a large bowl combine the cream cheese, artichoke, spinach and shredded cheeses.

Season with bouillon and salt and pepper to taste.

Pour into a shallow baking dish

Cover with GF bread crumbs

Bake for 20 minutes

Serve warm with crackers

This recipe would be great for a dinner party, football game or a girls night!

Best Gluten Free Bread Mixes

9th Annual Gluten-Free Awards:

1st Place Winner: Bob's Red Mill - Homemade Wonderful Bread Mix

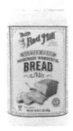

2nd Place Winner: Pamela's Products Gluten-free Bread Mix

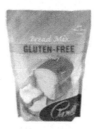

3rd Place Winner: gfJules Bread Mix

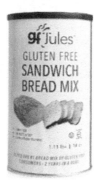

Other Great Products:

Chebe Bread Mix

Simple Mills Artisan Bread Mix

Luce's Gluten Free Artisan Bread Mix

Best Gluten Free Breakfast On-The-Go

9th Annual Gluten-Free Awards:

1st Place Winner: Pamela's Products Gluten Free Whenever Bars, Oat Chocolate Chip Coconut

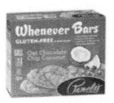

2nd Place Winner: Garden Lites Blueberry Blueberry Oat Muffins

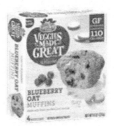

3rd Place Winner: Enjoy Life Seed and Fruit Mix

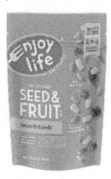

Other Great Products:

Amy's Tofu Scramble Breakfast Wrap, Gluten free

Bobo's Bar (Coconut)

thinkThin, Protein & Probiotics Hot Oatmeal

Wild Zora Paleo Meals To Go - Butte Cacao Banana

Mindy's Famous Gluten Free Cinnamon Rolls Recipe

Author: Jules Shepard

Prep Time: 30 minutes prep + 30 minutes rise

Cook Time: 12 minutes

Total Time: 1 hour 15 minutes

Yield: 12 rolls

Ingredients

(1/2 recipe measurements noted)

Rolls

1 cup+ (1/2 cup+ 3 Tbs.) warm water

3/4 – 1 cup (1/2 cup) room temp buttermilk (or non-dairy milk with 1/2 Tbs. lemon juice or white vinegar added)

1/2 cup (1/4 cup) sugar

1/4 cup (2 Tbs) melted butter (or vegan butter like Earth Balance® Buttery Sticks)

3 Tbs (1 packet – 2 1/4 tsp.) quick rise OR regular (GF) yeast (like Red Star® or Fleischmann's®) (Jules' note: do not use Red Star® Platinum yeast, as it is not gluten-free)

1/2 Tbs (1 tsp) salt

2 eggs (1 egg – or replacement like 1 Tbs. flaxseed meal steeped in 3 Tbs. warm water)

5 1/2 cups (742 grams) (2 3/4 cup or 371 grams) gf Jules™ Gluten Free All Purpose Flour

Filling

2 Tbs butter, melted (1 1/2 Tbs) (or vegan butter like Earth Balance® Buttery Sticks)

1/2 cup (1/4 cup) brown sugar

1/2 cup (1/4 cup) sugar

2 Tbs (1 Tbs) cinnamon

Frosting

1/4 cup (2 Tbs) butter, softened (or vegan butter like Earth Balance® Buttery Sticks)

3 cups (1 1/2 cups) sifted powdered sugar

1 tsp (1/2 tsp) pure vanilla extract

enough milk to make spreading consistency

dried cranberries or raisins (optional)

Instructions

Mix together water, buttermilk, sugar, melted butter and yeast in a bowl. If using quick rise yeast, allow to sit for 5 minutes; if using regular yeast, allow to sit for 15 minutes. The mixture should be frothy at this point, if not, discard and start over because the yeast is not active.

Add in salt, eggs and gfJules™ flour. (Jules Note: I added extra liquid, as noted in the ingredients, in order to get the dough to be more soft and pliable.) Mix for ten minutes (we use a Kitchenaid® mixer with the bread paddle attachment). Allow to sit for ten minutes. (Jules Note: I mixed only until ingredients were integrated and the dough was soft. Over-mixing gluten free dough may make it tough. I also did not allow it to sit after mixing but rolled the dough out immediately.)

While it is resting, prepare your filling by mixing together melted butter, brown sugar, sugar, and cinnamon.

Roll dough out onto a greased countertop into a 12×16 inch square or less, depending. (Jules Note: I rolled the dough onto a surface floured with gfJules™ Flour). Knowing that the dough will rise, roll the dough thinner if you prefer less bun and more filling, or the other way around!

Roll the dough before cutting — it will be close to the size of a rolling pin when rolled.

Spread filling and roll up. Cut into 12 rolls (6 -9 if making a 1/2 recipe).

Place rolls on cookie sheet covered with parchment paper or into an oiled baking pan. Allow to rise in a warm location for 30 minutes.

Bake at 400°F for 12-15 minutes. (Jules Note: I baked at 325° F for 12 minutes, or until a toothpick inserted into the rolls came out with only some dry crumbs.)

Remove to cool for a few minutes before whisking together frosting and drizzling on warm rolls.

Best Gluten Free Brownie Mix

9th Annual Gluten-Free Awards:

1st Place Winner: King Arthur Flour Gluten Free Brownie Mix

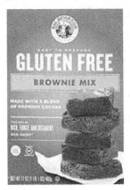

2nd Place Winner: Glutino Brownie Mix

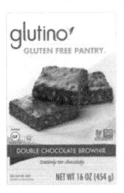

3rd Place Winner: Better Batter Gluten Free Fudge Brownie Mix

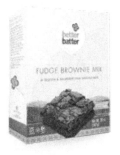

Other Great Products:

Namaste Gluten Free Brownie Mix

Enjoy Life Brownie Mix

Living Now - Chocolate Fudge Brownie Mix, Organic & Gluten-Free

Best Gluten Free Buns

9th Annual Gluten-Free Awards:

1st Place Winner: Udi's Gluten Free Classic Hamburger Buns

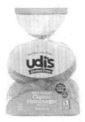

2nd Place Winner: Canyon Bakehouse Gluten Free Hamburger Buns

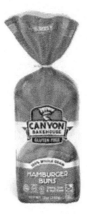

3rd Place Winner: Schar Gluten Free Hamburger Buns

Other Great Products:

Walmart "Sam's Choice" Private Label Gluten Free Hamburger Buns

Three Bakers' Whole Grain Hamburger Buns

Three Bakers' Whole Grain Hot Dog Buns

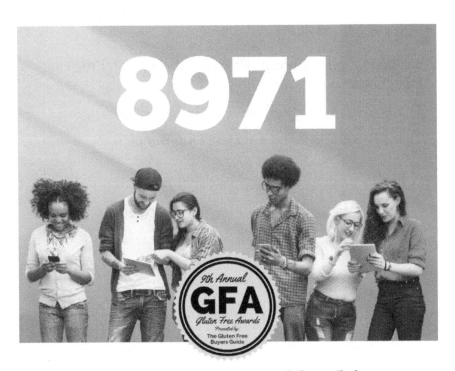

8,971 people voted in this years Gluten Free Awards.

Best Gluten Free Cake Mix

9th Annual Gluten-Free Awards:

1st Place Winner: Betty Crocker Gluten Free Yellow Cake Mix

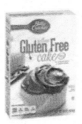

2nd Place Winner: King Arthur's Gluten Free Chocolate Cake Mix

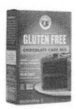

3rd Place Winner: King Arthur's Gluten Free Yellow Cake Mix

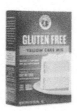

Other Great Products:

Better Batter Gluten Free Chocolate Cake Mix

Better Batter Gluten Free Yellow Cake Mix

Simple Mills Vanilla Cupcake & Cake Mix

The Really Great Food Company Gluten Free Coffee Crumb Cake Mix

Buddy's Allergen Free (Mug Cake) Chocolate Fudge with Chocolate Fudge Frosting

Best Gluten Free Children's Book

9th Annual Gluten-Free Awards:

1st Place Winner: Eat Like a Dinosaur: Recipe & Guidebook for Gluten-free Kids by Paleo Parents and Elana Amsterdam

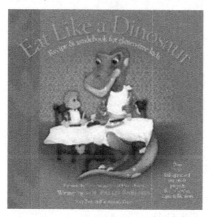

2nd Place Winner: The GF Kid: A Celiac Disease Survival Guide by Melissa London and Eric Glickman

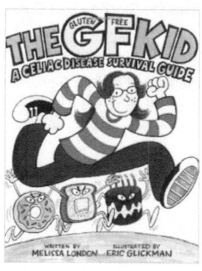

3rd Place Winner: Eating Gluten-Free with Emily: A Story for Children with Celiac Disease by Bonnie J. Kruszka and Richard S. Cihlar

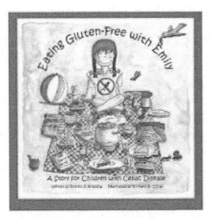

Other Great Products:

Adam's Gluten Free Surprise: Helping Others Understand Gluten Free by Debbie Simpson

Aidan the Wonder Kid Who Could Not Be Stopped: A Food Allergy and Intolerance Story by Dan Carsten and Colleen Brunetti

The Gluten Glitch by Stasie John and Kevin Cannon

Gordy and the Magic Diet by Kim Diersen (Author), April Runge (Author), Carrie Hartman (Illustrator)

Best Gluten Free Chips

9th Annual Gluten-Free Awards:

1st Place Winner: UTZ - Ripple Potato Chips

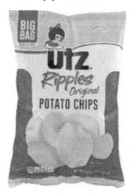

2nd Place Winner: Cape Cod Waffle Cut Chips

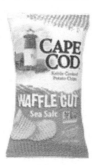

3rd Place Winner: Late July Snacks - Organic Multigrain Tortilla Chips Gluten Free Sea Salt By The Seashore

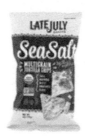

Other Great Products:

POPCORNERS Carnival Kettle, Popped Corn Chips, Gluten Free, Non-GMO

Enjoy Life Foods - Plentils, Sea Salt Lentil Chips

Way Better Snacks Sprouted Gluten Free Tortilla Chips Unbeatable Blues

Boulder Canyon - Coconut Oil Pineapple Habanero

Beanfields Bean and Rice Chips - Nacho

Best Gluten Free Cold Cereal

9th Annual Gluten-Free Awards:

1st Place Winner: Cinnamon Rice Chex

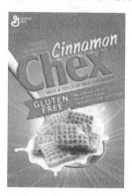

2nd Place Winner: Post Cocoa Pebbles

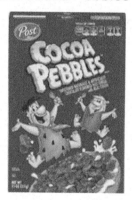

3rd Place Winner: Envirokidz Panda Puffs

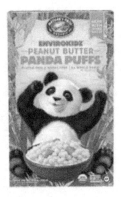

Other Great Products:

Nature's Path Amazon Flakes

Love Grown Fruity Sea Stars

Freedom Foods Tropico's

Best Gluten Free Accommodating Colleges

9th Annual Gluten-Free Awards:

1st Place Winner: UNIVERSITY OF CALIFORNIA, LOS ANGELES

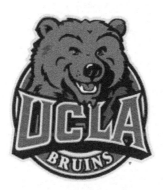

2nd Place Winner: UNIVERSITY OF COLORADO: BOULDER

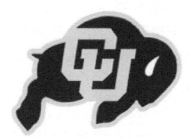

3rd Place Winner: UNIVERSITY OF NOTRE DAME

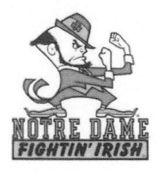

Other Great Schools:

NC STATE UNIVERSITY

UNIVERSITY OF TENNESSEE

KENT STATE UNIVERSITY

YALE UNIVERSITY

OREGON STATE UNIVERSITY

UNIVERSITY OF NEW HAMPSHIRE

UNIVERSITY OF ARIZONA

IOWA STATE UNIVERSITY

ITHACA COLLEGE

UNIVERSITY OF CONNECTICUT

SAN DIEGO STATE

GEORGETOWN UNIVERSITY

COLUMBIA UNIVERSITY

TOWSON UNIVERSITY

CLARK UNIVERSITY

CARLETON COLLEGE

Best Gluten Free Comfort Food

9th Annual Gluten-Free Awards:

1st Place Winner: Amy's Gluten Free Frozen Mac and Cheese

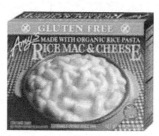

2nd Place Winner: Annie's Gluten Free Rice Pasta & Cheddar

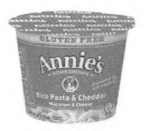

3rd Place Winner: Udi's Meal Mac & Cheese Bakeable Meal

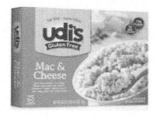

Other Great Products:

ALDI: liveGfree Gluten Free Chicken Breast Nuggets

Lundberg Creamy Parmesan Risotto

Gratify - Cinnamon Baked Bites

Free 2 Be - Rice Chocolate Sun Cups

Best Gluten Free Cookbooks

9th Annual Gluten-Free Awards:

1st Place Winner: Gluten-Free on a Shoestring: 125 Easy Recipes for Eating Well on the Cheap by Nicole Hunn

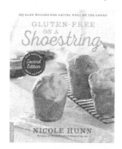

2nd Place Winner : The How Can It Be Gluten Free Cookbook: Revolutionary Techniques. Groundbreaking Recipes by America's Test Kitchen

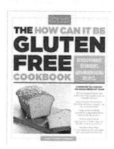

3rd Place Winner: Free for All Cooking: 150 Easy Gluten-Free, Allergy-Friendly Recipes the Whole Family Can Enjoy by Jules E. Dowler Shepard

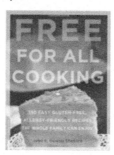

Other Great Products:

Nearly Normal Cooking For Gluten-Free Eating: A Fresh Approach to Cooking and Living Without Wheat or Gluten by Jules E. D. Shepard and Alessio Fasano

1,000 Gluten-Free Recipes (1,000 Recipes) by Carol Fenster

Danielle Walker's Against All Grain Celebrations: A Year of Gluten-Free, Dairy-Free, and Paleo Recipes for Every Occasion by Danielle Walker

The Easy Gluten-Free Cookbook: Fast and Fuss-Free Recipes for Busy People on a Gluten-Free Diet by Lindsay Garza

The Gluten Free Cookbook for Families: Healthy Recipes in 30 Minutes or Lessby Pamela Ellgen and Alice Bast

The Big Book of Gluten Free Cooking: Delicious Meals, Breads, and Sweets for a Happy, Healthy Gluten-Free Lifeby Gigi Stewart B.S. M.A.

Sweet & Simple Gluten-Free Baking: Irresistible Classics in 10 Ingredients or Less! by Chrystal Carver

Eat Happy: Gluten Free, Grain Free, Low Carb Recipes For A Joyful Life by Anna Vocino

Bread & Butter: Gluten-Free Vegan Recipes to Fill Your Bread Basket by Erin McKenna

Pure Fresh Donuts by Lori Miller

DID YOU KNOW?

CELIAC DISEASE: INCREASED TO 3% IN US (NOT 1% AS CONSISTENTLY REPORTED)

Quoted from:
17th International Celiac Disease
Symposium in New Delhi, India

5 Lies We Tell About Our Food Allergy Issues

Erica Dermer, author of Celiac and the Beast: A Love Story between a Gluten-Free Girl, Her Genes and a Broken Digestive Tract.

"This article originally appeared in Gluten Free & More Magazine."

Let's be honest. People with celiac disease and gluten sensitivity are pretenders. We tell tales to make our lives (and other people's) easier. In the long run, however, facing—and speaking—the truth is better for us and for those we're with. Here's the scoop on the top five fibs we tell...and how to come clean.

5 Reasons Why We Lie about our Food Allergy Issues

Lie #1

"I'm not hungry."

It can be annoying to repeat your gluten-free speech to strangers. Sometimes it's just easier to say you're not hungry than explain you're not comfortable eating food you didn't make yourself. (All this while you're eyeballing that cake in the corner like it's the last dessert on earth!)

The Truth It's okay to say you're avoiding certain foods. Create a short and simple "elevator speech," lasting no longer than a brief elevator ride. Learn to clearly communicate your food needs within 30 seconds.

Lie #2

"I'm sure it's safe."

Sometimes people on a gluten-free diet convince themselves that a suspect food item is safe, thus engaging in risky behavior. Maybe you're at a Mexican restaurant and you grab a handful of tortilla chips, assuming they're safe—

but mostly because you want to snack like everyone else. The chips could have been prepared in the same fryer as gluten-containing foods.

The Truth Don't take chances by assuming anything. Always ask, even if you're afraid it may be embarrassing. Put your safety first.

Lie #3

"This is good."

The number of gluten-free options has grown by leaps and bounds in the last five years. The choices are abundant. We can buy gluten-free breads, pastas and baked goods at almost any grocery store. But while much of it tastes terrific, not all of it is great.

The Truth Let's not settle. Never stop hunting for the safest and most delicious versions of your favorite gluten-full foods. Support businesses that work hard to refine their product lines to be the best they can be. Make sure the products are certified gluten-free and made in a dedicated facility or on dedicated equipment.

Lie #4

"I'm allergic to gluten."

You don't want to stand out, right? So you adapt your language to fit the overall culture—and "allergy" and "gluten" are very familiar terms to most people and to those in the food industry. But celiac disease and gluten intolerance are not food allergies. Celiac disease is an autoimmune disease that is provoked by gluten contained in wheat, rye, barley, contaminated oats and their derivatives.

The Truth Try to be accurate while keeping it simple. Here's a quick way to get the point across: "I have celiac disease and gluten makes me very sick."

Lie #5

"I'm OK."

How many times have you told someone you're okay when you're not? We're used to hiding our true emotions. With the barrage of gluten-free jokes in the media and the lack of respect from some around us, it's challenging to admit when we're not feeling so great or doing so well. Besides, we don't want to bore others with our food issues, right?

The Truth It's okay to tell a friend you're not okay. It's okay to feel frustrated and to vent. Find a trusted group of people like you—at an expo, support group or online community—and you'll be able to safely share with others how you really feel. And that feels good.

Managing editor Erica Dermer (edermer@glutenfreeandmore.com) is author of Celiac and the Beast: A Love Story between a Gluten-Free Girl, Her Genes and a Broken Digestive Tract.

Best Gluten Free Cookie Mixes

9th Annual Gluten-Free Awards:

1st Place Winner: Betty Crocker Gluten Free Cookie Mix Chocolate Chip

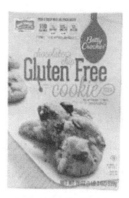

2nd Place Winner: Pamela's Products Gluten Free Cookie Mix, Chocolate Chunk

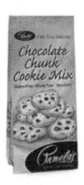

3rd Place Winner gfJules Cookie Mix

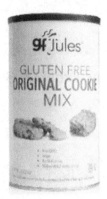

Other Great Products:

Immaculate Baking Gluten Free Cookie Mix Sugar

Hodgson Mill Gluten Free Cookie Mix

Simple Mills Chocolate Chip Cookie

Sweet Loren's Place & Bake Gluten Free Chocolate Chunk

Best Gluten Free Cookies

9th Annual Gluten-Free Awards:

1st Place Winner: Tate's Chocolate Chip

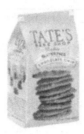

2nd Place Winner: Enjoy Life Foods | Soft Baked Snickerdoodle Mini Cookies

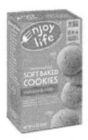

3rd Place Winner: Schär: Chocolate Dipped Cookies

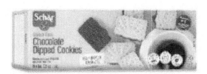

Other Great Products:

Trader Joe's Joe Joes

Lucy's Gluten-free Sugar Cookies

Aleia's Almond Horns

Three Bakers' Chocolate Chip Snackers

Three Bakers' Chocolate Chocolate Chip Snackers

Cybele's Free to Eat Chocolate Chip Cookies

Laughing Giraffe Organics Lemon Snakaroons

Laughing Giraffe Organics Chocolate Snakaroons

Best Gluten Free Cornbread Mix

9th Annual Gluten-Free Awards:

1st Place Winner: Krusteaz Gluten Free Cornbread Mix

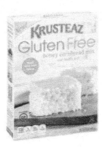

2nd Place Winner: Bob's Red Mill Gluten Free Cornbread Mix

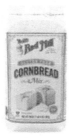

3rd Place Winner: gfJules Cornbread Mix

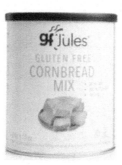

Other Great Products:

Pamela's Gluten Free Cornbread Mix

Glutino Cornbread Mix

Gluten Free Pantry Cornbread Muffin Mix Wheat Free

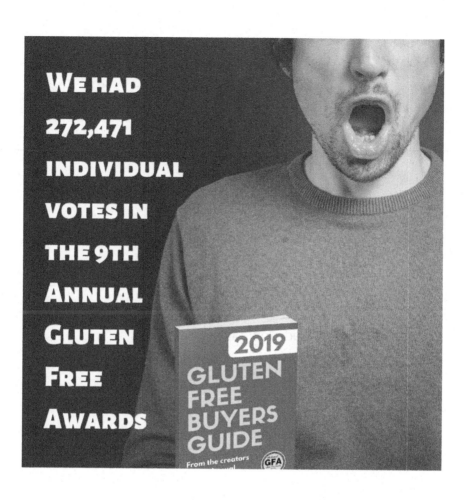

We had 272,471 individual votes in the 9th Annual Gluten Free Awards

Best Gluten Free Cosmetic Brands

9th Annual Gluten-Free Awards:

1st Place Winner: tarte

tarte
high-performance naturals˜

2nd Place Winner: Arbonne

ℬ ARBONNE.

3rd Place Winner: Red Apple Lipstick

red apple lipstick
gluten free, paraben free : safe

Other Great Products:

Au Naturale

Afterglow

Kiss Freely

Gabriel Cosmetics

ILIA Beauty

Best Gluten Free Crackers

9th Annual Gluten-Free Awards:

1st Place Winner: Schär Table Crackers

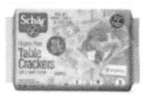

2nd Place Winner: Milton's Gluten Free Cheddar Cheese Crackers

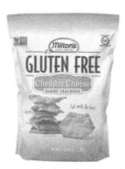

3rd Place Winner: Trader Joe's Rice Crackers

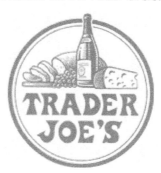

Other Great Products:

Simple Mills Fine Ground Sea Salt Almond Flour Crackers

Simple Mills Almond Flour Crackers

Gratify Original Baked Bites

Best Gluten Free Donuts

9th Annual Gluten-Free Awards:

1st Place Winner: Katz Gluten Free, Glazed Donuts

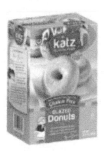

2nd Place Winner: Kinnikinnick Gluten Free Vanilla Glazed Donut

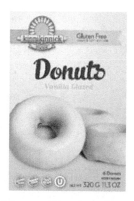

3rd Place Winner: Katz Gluten Free, Glazed Chocolate Donut Holes

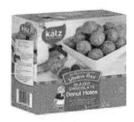

Other Great Products:

Katz Gluten Free, Powdered Donut

Kinnikinnick Gluten Free Maple Glazed Donut

KNOW Better Donuts

Best Gluten Free Expo and Events

9th Annual Gluten-Free Awards:

1st Place Winner: Gluten & Allergen Free Expos

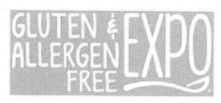

2nd Place Winner: Living Without's Gluten Free Food Allergy Fest

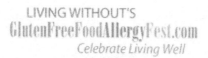

3rd Place Winner: Gluten & Allergen Free Wellness Events

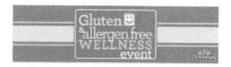

Other Great Gluten Free Expos:

CDF National Education & Gluten-Free Expo

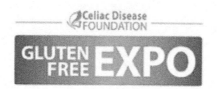

Natural Products Expo West

Natural Products Expo East

Best Gluten Free Flours

9th Annual Gluten-Free Awards:

1st Place Winner: Bob's Red Mill Gluten Free 1-to-1 Baking Flour

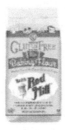

2nd Place Winner: King Arthur Gluten Free Flour

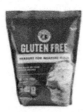

3rd Place Winner: gfJules All Purpose Gluten Free Flour

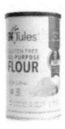

Other Great Products:

Better Batter Gluten Free Flour, cup for cup

Cup 4 Cup™ Gluten Free Flour Blend

Glutino Gluten-Free Pantry All Purpose Baking Flour

Namaste Perfect Flour Blend

Enjoy Life All-Purpose Flour

Lidl Gluten Free Flour Mix

Gluten-Free Prairie Simply Wholesome All Purpose Flour Blend

Terrasoul Superfoods - Cassava Flour

The Best Gluten Free Cake Recipe

Author: Jules Shepard

Prep Time: 15 minutes

Cook Time: 30 minutes + 15 minute rest

Total Time: 1 hour

Yield: 1 round cake or 12 cupcakes

Ingredients

Note: double for two 8 or 9-inch round pans

- 1 ½ cups (202.5 grams) gfJules™ All Purpose Gluten Free Flour
- 1 cup minus 1 Tbs. granulated cane sugar
- 2 tsp. baking powder
- 1/3 tsp. baking soda
- 2 eggs or substitute (for white cake, use 4 egg whites instead)
- 1/3 cup mild flavored vegetable oil of choice (safflower, non-GMO canola, extra virgin olive oil, coconut oil melted, etc.)
- 1 Tbs. white vinegar
- 1 tsp. pure vanilla extract (I like Rodelle®)
- ½ cup milk of choice (dairy or non-dairy; skim or fat-free not recommended)

For Chocolate Cake, add ¼ cup cocoa, ¼ cup additional milk and 3 tablespoons chocolate syrup (I like Ah!Laska® Organic Dairy Free Syrup).

Instructions

Preheat oven to 350° F.

Oil one 8 or 9-inch round cake pan or line 12 muffin cups with cupcake papers.

Bring all ingredients to room temperature. Sift the dry ingredients together in a bowl. In a separate mixing bowl, combine liquid ingredients, reserving milk. Slowly pour dry mix into the liquids and begin to stir, adding the milk while stirring to keep the flour from flying up and out of the bowl while mixing. Continue to beat at medium speed just until the lumps are gone and the batter is smooth.

Pour batter into prepared pan(s). Allow to rest in the pan before baking for 15 minutes.

Bake for approximately 30-35 minutes for the cake and 20-25 minutes for the cupcakes. Test with a toothpick before removing from the oven. When done, the toothpick should come out clean (not wet), and may have a few crumbs attached when inserted into the center of the cake. Glass, metal and ceramic pans all alter the bake time, so check for done-ness before removing from the oven.

Remove to cool on a wire rack. To remove the cake, gently invert the cake by flipping it upside down onto your hand, removing the pan, then returning the cake to the wire rack or a serving plate.

Notes

Frost with your favorite frosting like this white or chocolate frosting recipe. (There are plenty more frosting recipes where that came from – just search the "recipes" tab on my site!)

Best Gluten Free Frozen Meals

9th Annual Gluten-Free Awards:

1st Place Winner: Amy's Rice Macaroni & Cheese, Gluten-Free

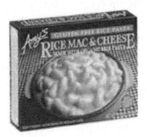

2nd Place Winner: Udi's Broccoli and Kale Lasagna

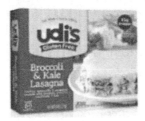

3rd Place Winner: Evol Fire Grilled Steak Bowl

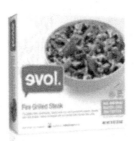

Other Great Products:

Gluten Free Delights - Uncured Pepperoni Pizza

Amy's Chinese Noodles & Veggies in Cashew Cream Sauce

Feel Good Foods Entree Mongolian Beef with Asparagus

Gluten Free Delights - Ham & Cheese

Luvo Hawaiian Un-Fried Rice

Best Gluten Free Frozen Pancake & Waffle Brands

9th Annual Gluten-Free Awards:

1st Place Winner: Van's Gluten Free Waffles

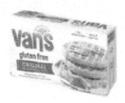

2nd Place Winner: Trader Joe's Gluten-Free Waffles

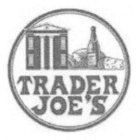

3rd Place Winner: Nature's Path Homestyle Frozen Waffle

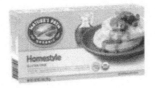

Other Great Products:

Kashi Gluten Free Waffles

Know Foods Gluten Free Waffles

Best Gluten Free Frozen Pizza Brands

9th Annual Gluten-Free Awards:

1st Place Winner: Udi's Gluten Free Pepperoni Pizza

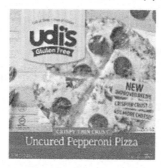

2nd Place Winner: California Pizza Kitchen Gluten Free BBQ Chicken

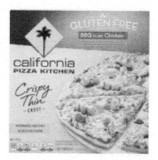

3rd Place Winner: Against the Grain Nut-Free Pesto Pizza

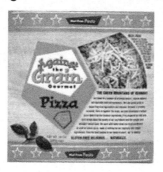

Other Great Products:

Amy's Gluten Free Cheese Pizza

Sabatasso's Gluten Free Four Cheese Pizza

Sonoma Flatbread Uncured Pepperoni

Three Bakers' Cheese Pizza

Three Bakers' Pepperoni Pizza

Three Bakers' Italian Sausage Pizza

Oggi Foods Inc. : Cauliflower Pizza Crust

Oggi Foods Inc. : Margherita Pizza

DID YOU KNOW?

GLUTEN CAN'T BE DIGESTED BY HUMAN BODY (LONG CHAIN AMINO ACID)

Quoted from:
17th International Celiac Disease
Symposium in New Delhi, India

Best Gluten Free Granola

9th Annual Gluten-Free Awards:

1st Place Winner: Udi's Au Naturel Gluten Free Granola, Wildflower Honey Oats

2nd Place Winner: Bakery On Main's Gluten-Free, Non GMO Granola, Cranberry Almond Maple

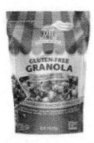

3rd Place Winner: ALDI: liveGfree Gluten Free Granola - Cranberry Cashew

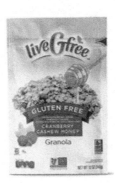

Other Great Products:

ALDI: liveGfree Gluten Free Granola - Apple Almond Honey

ALDI: liveGfree Gluten Free Granola - Raisin Almond Honey

Purely Elizabeth Ancient Grain Granola, Original

Bubba's Fine Foods Bourbon Vanilla UnGranola

Goodness Grainless Granola Chocolate Cardamom

Autumn's Gold Grain Free Granola

Lidl Organic, Gluten Free Crunchy Granola

Best Gluten Free Ice Cream Cones

9th Annual Gluten-Free Awards:

1st Place Winner: Edward & Sons Trading Co. Ice Cream Cones, Gluten Free

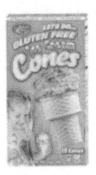

2nd Place Winner: Goldbaum's Gluten Free Ice Cream Cone

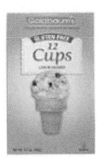

3rd Place Winner: Edward & Sons Trading Co. Cones, Sugar, Gluten Free

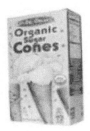

Other Great Products:

Barkat Gluten Free Waffle Ice Cream Cones

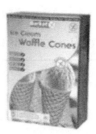

Best Gluten Free Jerky

9th Annual Gluten-Free Awards:

1st Place Winner: Oberto Original Beef Jerky

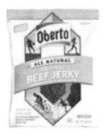

2nd Place Winner: Krave Sweet Chipotle Beef Jerky

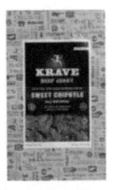

3rd Place Winner: EPIC Bison and Bacon Bites

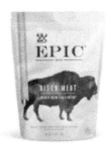

Other Great Products:

Country Archer Grass Fed Original Beef Jerky

Krave Pineapple Orange Beef Jerky

Oberto Spicy Sweet Beef Jerky

EPIC Cranberry Sriracha Beef Bites

Be apart of our
10th Anniversary

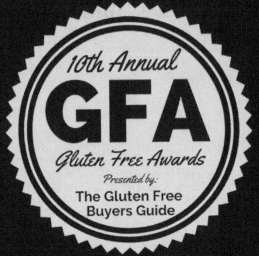

Register Now

Best Gluten Free Macaroni and Cheese

9th Annual Gluten-Free Awards:

1st Place Winner: Amy's Gluten Free Frozen Mac & Cheese

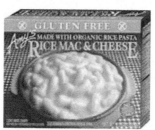

2nd Place Winner: Annie's Organic Vegan Macaroni and Cheese, Elbows & Creamy Sauce, Gluten Free Pasta

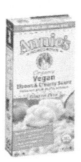

3rd Place Winner: ALDI: liveGfree Gluten Free Deluxe Macaroni & Cheese

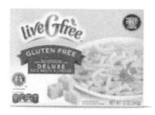

Other Great Products:

Trader Joe's Gluten Free Mac & Cheese

Udi's Buffalo Style Chicken Mac & Cheese

Lidl Gluten Free Macaroni and Cheese Assortment

Homemade Spaghetti O's (Allergy-Free, Gluten-Free, Vegan)

Rebecca Pytell, creator of Strength and Sunshine (https://strengthandsunshine.com)

Kick the can and make this healthy recipe for the kids instead! Homemade Spaghetti O's that are allergy-free, gluten-free, and vegan! A super easy lunch or dinner that's kid-friendly and mom-approved!

Guys, SPAGHETTI O'S! An American childhood classic, am I right? Thick, creamy, tomatoey pasta in a can. All condensed with artificial colors, preservatives, flavors, BPA, sugars, salt, fat, and a bunch of other scary things! There's 600mg of sodium and 11g of sugar in just a 1 cup serving! Ah! Not only should the terrible nutrition cause you fear, but the lack of food allergy safety (obviously). Every child should experience Spaghetti O's, but we can clean it up a bit (or a lot) and make it so much better for all!

My brother was more of the Spaghetti O's eater in the house, but I did eat it back in the day. One day last summer, I felt compelled to recreate this processed meal-in-a-can to be healthy and allergy-free. It's hard to explain the taste, texture, and consistency of Spaghetti O's, so I had some work to do to make this homemade version just right. Since I can't even remember a ballpark range of the last time I had the "goods", I ended up doing some tastebud memory digging and online research!

I also had "the fam" to be my taste-testers too! If you have some gluten-free eaters or other food allergy (like dairy) child running around in your house and you don't want them to miss out on this, you don't have to feel bad! Or, maybe you're like me, a bustling busy millennial and you still crave childhood favorites from time to time. You don't have to crack open a can of cold Spaghetti O's and eat it straight up like the stereotypical "college diet" calls for. You can make some delicious and nutritious Homemade Spaghetti O's super quick, in one pot, and worthy of being served to guests as well!

You might not believe me, but these taste spot-on! The thick consistency of the "cheesy" creamy tomato sauce and those soft little Os! Healthy and allergy-free "junk food"? I always have you covered! This recipe for Homemade Spaghetti O's is so easy and with minimal and "no weird" ingredients! Just cook the gluten-free pasta, drain, throw it back in the pot, and add the sauce ingredients! You'll be eating Homemade Spaghetti O's for days! Your kids and yourself, for work and school, grab a handy thermos and take the goods with you, cold or hot!

Cook time

10 mins

Total time

10 mins

Author: Rebecca Pytell

Recipe type: Main

Cuisine: American

Serves: 4-6

Ingredients

1 (12oz) Box Gluten-Free Anellini Pasta

1 (15oz) Can No-Salt Added Tomato Sauce

⅓ Cup Unsweetened Non-Dairy Milk

¼ Cup Nutritional Yeast

2 TB Tomato Paste

1 Tsp Onion Powder

½ Tsp Garlic Powder

½ Tsp Paprika

Instructions

In a large pot, cook pasta according to box directions, drain, and add back into pot.

Now add all other ingredients to the pot, with heat turned to low and mix well to combine.

Serve warm or cold!

Nutrition Information

Serving size: 1

Who said Spaghetti O's weren't healthy, wholesome, and nutritious? That's right...I did...but HOMEMADE Spaghetti O's are! Don't you just love it when that happens? I don't know about you, but these make me feel all warm and cozy! We allergy-free, gluten-free, vegan eaters don't let anything get in our way for devouring our old favorite foods (in a new, healthy, modern way)! Now, let's get cooking!

Best Gluten Free Magazines

9th Annual Gluten-Free Awards:

1st Place Winner: Gluten-Free Living

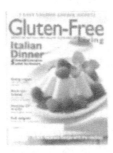

2nd Place Winner: Simply Gluten Free

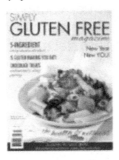

3rd Place Winner: Living Without's Gluten Free & More

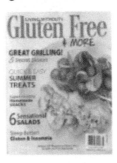

Other Great Products:

Delight Gluten Free

GFF Magazine

Allergic Living

yum.

Gluten Free Globalicious Magazine

Best Gluten Free Mobile Apps

9th Annual Gluten-Free Awards:

1st Place Winner: Find Me Gluten Free

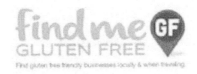

2nd Place Winner: The Gluten Free Scanner

3rd Place Winner: Epicurious

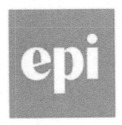

Other Great Apps:

ShopWell

Grain or No Grain

Best Gluten Free Muffin Mix

9th Annual Gluten-Free Awards:

1st Place Winner: King Arthur Gluten Free Muffin Mix

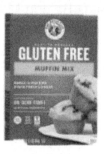

2nd Place Winner: gfJules Muffin Mix

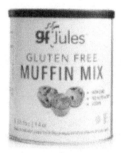

3rd Place Winner: Enjoy Life Muffin Mix

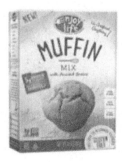

Other Great Products:

Namaste Foods Gluten Free Muffin Mix

Simple Mills Naturally Gluten-Free Almond Flour Mix, Pumpkin Muffin & Bread

Bona Dea Ancient Grains Baking Mix Muffins

Best Gluten Free Munchies

9th Annual Gluten-Free Awards:

1st Place Winner: Glutino Yogurt Covered Pretzels

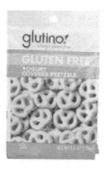

2nd Place Winner: Cape Cod Waffle Cut Sea Salt Chips

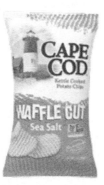

3rd Place Winner: Three Bakers' Honey Graham Snackers

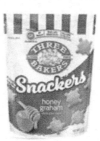

Other Great Products:

Three Bakers' Real Cheddar Snackers

Popcornopolis Zebra Corn

Bobo's Bites - Bobo's Chocolate Chip Bites

The Good Bean Sea Salt Chickpeas

Epic Brand Pork Rinds - Sea Salt and Pepper

Bubba's Fine Foods Savory Original Snack Mix

The Good Bean Balsamic Herb Favas + Peas

The Good Bean Habenero Citrus Favas + Peas

Best Gluten Free National Restaurant Chains

9th Annual Gluten-Free Awards:

1st Place Winner: Red Robin

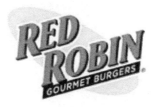

2nd Place Winner: P.F. Chang's

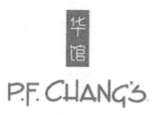

3rd Place Winner: Chipotle

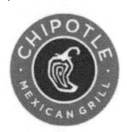

Other Great Products:

Outback Steakhouse

The Bonefish Grill

Jersey Mike's

True Food Kitchen

The Counter – Custom Burgers

Best Gluten Free New Products

9th Annual Gluten-Free Awards:

1st Place Winner: Udi's Gluten Free Delicious Bread Soft White

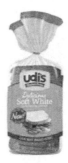

2nd Place Winner: Canyon Bakehouse Original English Muffins

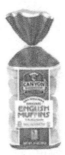

3rd Place Winner: Udi's Gluten Free Delicious Bread Multigrain

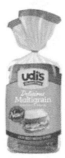

Other Great Products:

Enjoy Life Foods | Dipped Banana Protein Bites

Bobo's Stuff'd Bars - Bobo's Peanut Butter Stuff'd Chocolate Chip

thinkThin, Protein Cakes

The Good Bean Sea Salt Grab-N'-Go Snacks

The Maple Guild – Organic Maple Butter

The Maple Guild – Organic Bourbon Barrel Aged Syrup

The Good Bean Sweet Sriarcha Grab-N'-Go Snacks

The Maple Guild – Organic Maple Vinegar

Best Gluten Free Non-Profits

9th Annual Gluten-Free Awards:

1st Place Winner: Celiac Disease Foundation (CDF)

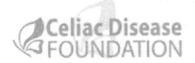

2nd Place Winner: Gluten Intolerance Group of North America (GIG)

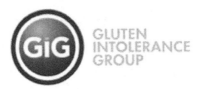

3rd Place Winner: Celiac Support Association

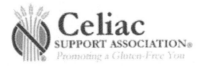

Other Great Non-Profits:

National Celiac Disease Society (NCDS)

Beyond Celiac

Cutting Costs for Celiacs Food Equality Initiative

DID YOU KNOW?

1:2 IN THE UNITED STATES WILL TRY A GLUTEN-FREE DIET THIS YEAR

Quoted from:
17th International Celiac Disease
Symposium in New Delhi, India

Best Gluten Free Online Resources

9th Annual Gluten-Free Awards:

1st Place Winner: Celiac.org

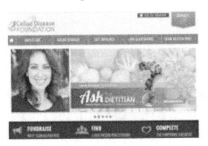

2nd Place Winner: GlutenFreeWatchDog.org

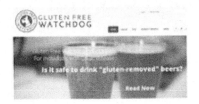

3rd Place Winner: Beyondceliac.org

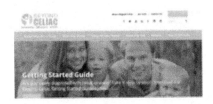

Other Great Websites:

Celiac.com

Gluten.org

CeliacCentral.org

Best Gluten Free Online Stores

9th Annual Gluten-Free Awards:

1st Place Winner: Amazon

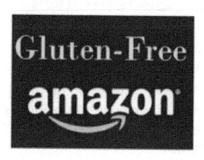

2nd Place Winner: Gluten Free Mall

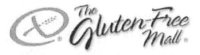

3rd Place Winner: Thrive Market

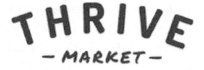

Other Great Stores:

Vitacost

Walmart Online

Target Online

Nuts.com

Jet.com

Gluten Free, Dairy Free Travel Guide: How to Survive a trip with Celiac, Food Allergies, or Sensitivities

Christina Kantzavelos, creator of BuenQamino (buenqamino.com)

Traveling with Celiac Disease or food sensitivities is something that can be anxiety provoking. However, with the right tools and resources, it is not only doable, but extremely enjoyable. Here's how...

1. Do Your Research

What is the food like where are you going? What are the general ingredients used in the traditional meals there? I like to research the cuisine, and find the plates that are naturally and unmistakingly allergen-free.

Are there gluten-free or allergen-friendly brands or restaurants in the country you're visitings? Are there grocery stores nearby where you are staying? I research Celiac and other Allergen-Friendly Associations to see what information they have posted (sometimes they even host gatherings!). I also like to look at other blogs that might have written posts on the country or City I am visiting.

I also research English-speaking hospitals and clinics in the area .... Just in case. This research will save you a lot of stress later on, and you can enjoy your trip with much less food related stress.

2. Carry a Translation Card for food allergies, drug allergies, diet restrictions

This is extremely helpful to carry around so that the person serving you food, or offering you any service is aware of your allergies or restrictions. The translation isn't a simple Google Translation, but rather put in terms the person from that country will understand. Also, no one wants to purposefully make your dining unpleasant, and this will take away the potential for much back and forth confusion. Keep in mind that you are their guest too.

I have food allergies...

3. Learn the Language

Unfortunately, not everyone is literate in this world (consider only 86% of us in the USA are). With that said, you may want to learn a phrase or two, or at least know how to say gluten, dairy or any other allergen items in that language. Plus, it's just nice. You can begin learning most languages for free using one of my favorite apps, Duolingo.

4. Medication(s), or other Supplements

I bring my EpiPen wherever I go, because I have a history of anaphylaxis. I also use Digestive Enzymes, and carry Activated Charcoal in case I accidentally ingest something I am allergic to, Benadryl in case I break out into hives, Excedrin for my fun migraines, Elemental Magesium for regularity, Methyl B12 for my MTHFR/energy, an inhaler for my seasonal asthma, and sodium/electrolyte supplements for my POTS. Bring what you need because medical help may not be readily available.

5. Mobile Applications and Website Resources

There are plenty of food apps and websites out there that will tell you where to find allergen-friendly food. I personally like to use Find Me Gluten Free and The Coeliac Plate, which both list gluten-free restaurants/venues in each city.

6. Grocery Shop

Get to know your local grocery store, wherever you're staying. You can buy whole foods to cook with, or to eat on the go. Sometimes, you might be surprised that they even have a gluten free or vegan section.

7. Private Kitchen

If it's possible to have access to your own kitchen in a place you're staying, whether that's AirBnB, or a hostel, then you are able to buy your own ingredients locally and cook yourself a meal. You can also pack a spatula, wooden spoon, and parchment paper for the pots and pans to avoid cross contamination. I have a great time using local whole ingredients to create healthy meals.

8. Carry Food Staples

Depending on the trip, I like to carry some staples with me. These include, but are not limited to:

Nutrition bars - These saved me on the Camino, and other trips. Sometimes it's difficult to get in the calories you need, and these help.

Sriracha - To spice things up. Wish I had brought this on the Camino!

GF soy sauce packets - Because it makes just about everything taste good, and it's harder to find abroad!

Rice Crackers - Easy to carry, dry and delicious!

Loaf of GF bread - I recommend this for shorter, and/or nearby trips. I sadly had mine squashed on flight to Iceland, and it looked like a framable footprint by the end of it.

9. Reusable Toaster / Grill Bags

These are great if you are staying in an AirBnB, hotel or visiting a cafe with a toaster, or grill. They prevent cross contamination! They are also great to toast or grill entire sandwiches in, holding all of the good stuff together.

10. Traveler's Insurance

My personal health insurance didn't work when I ended up in the hospital in Japan. If I had travel insurance, I would've been at least reimbursed for the amount I had to pay out of pocket. I now know, and do better thanks to World Nomads Travel Insurance. I recently used it when I was hospitalized in Mexico, and they not only reimbursed me for my hospital visit, but they also reimbursed me for having to travel back home earlier than expected.

Travel Insurance. Simple & Flexible.

Which countries or regions are you traveling to?

What's your country of residence?

Start date

End date

Enter Traveler's Age

Get a Price

11. Food Sensitivity Test

I like to be 100% sure that I am not consuming anything that will cause an instant or delayed sensitivity, or allergic reaction. This is why I recently purchased an at-home Food Sensitivity Test from EverlyWell, which measures your body's response to over 96 foods.

12. Let NIMA do the dirty work for you...

All hail science. NIMA is a portable gluten and peanut sensor that tests your food for you, before you decide to munch on it. Now you can always be sure!

Best Gluten Free Pancake and Waffle Mixes

9th Annual Gluten-Free Awards:

1st Place Winner: Bisquick Gluten Free

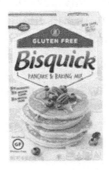

2nd Place Winner: Pamela's Products Gluten Free Baking and Pancake Mix

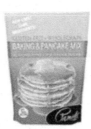

3rd Place Winner: gfJules Pancake & Waffle Mix

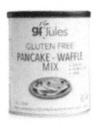

Other Great Products:

Better Batter Gluten Free Pancake and Biscuit Mix

Trader Joe's Gluten Free Buttermilk Pancake & Waffle Mix

Birch Benders Gluten Free Pancake & Waffle Mix

Gluten-Free Prairie Simply Our Best Pancake and Waffle Mix

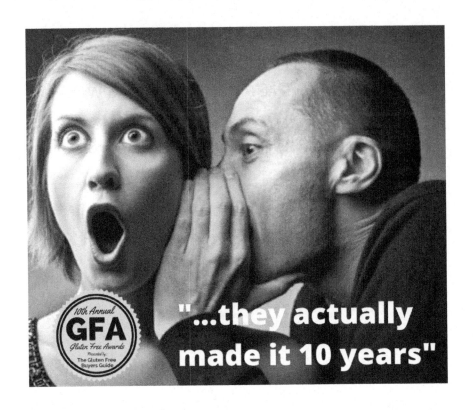

Best Gluten Free Pastas

9th Annual Gluten-Free Awards:

1st Place Winner: Barilla Gluten Free Rotini

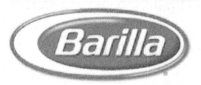

2nd Place Winner: Ronzoni Gluten Free Penne Rigate

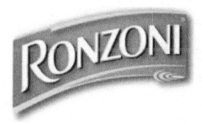

3rd Place Winner: Jovial Fusilli Gluten Free Pasta

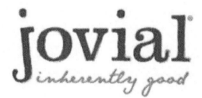

Other Great Products:

ALDI: liveGfree Gluten Free Brown Rice Spaghetti

ALDI: liveGfree Organic Gluten Free Brown Rice Quinoa - Penne Pasta

ALDI: liveGfree Organic Gluten Free Brown Rice Quinoa - Fusilli Pasta

Cappello's Gluten Free Fettuccine

Le Veneziane Fettucce

Le Veneziane Spaghetti

Lidl Gluten Free Penne

Lidl Gluten Free Spaghetti

Lidl Gluten Free Deluxe Pasta

Best Gluten Free Pie Crust

9th Annual Gluten-Free Awards:

1st Place Winner: King Arthur Flour Gluten Free Pie Crust Mix

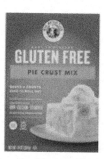

2nd Place Winner: Glutino Perfect Pie Crust Mix

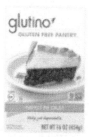

3rd Place Winner: Midel Graham Cracker Crust

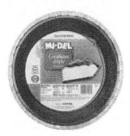

Other Great Products:

Cup4Cup Gluten-Free Pie Crust Mix

Williams Sonoma Gluten-Free Pie Crust Mix

Inspiration Mix Gluten Free Pie Crust Mix

Best Gluten Free Pizza Crust

9th Annual Gluten-Free Awards:

1st Place Winner: Bob's Red Mill Pizza Crust Mix

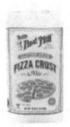

2nd Place Winner: gfJules Pizza Crust Mix

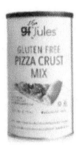

3rd Place Winner: Enjoy Life Pizza Crust Mix

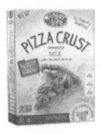

Other Great Products:

Three Bakers Traditional Thin Whole Grain Pizza Crust

Simple Mills Pizza Dough Mix

Cooqi Gluten Free Pizza & Pita Mix

Best Gluten Free Pretzels

9th Annual Gluten-Free Awards:

1st Place Winner: Snyder's of Hanover Gluten Free Pretzel Sticks

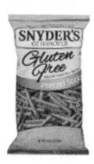

2nd Place Winner: Glutino Pretzel Twists, Salted

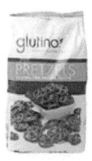

3rd Place Winner: ALDI liveGfree Pretzel Sticks

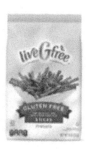

Other Great Products:

Schar Gluten Free Pretzels

Tonya's Gluten Free Soft Pretzels

Lidl Gluten Free Pretzel Assortment

Good Health Inc. Gluten Free Sea Salt Pretzels

Meatballs (Paleo, Gluten Free, Dairy Free,
Egg Free)

Jennifer Bigler, creator of Living Freely Gluten Free, LLC.

www.livingfreelyglutenfree.com

When I decided to write down my meatball recipe I knew I wanted to keep it simple. Not only did I want the meatballs to be gluten and dairy free, but I knew I could make an amazing tasting meatball that was naturally paleo. Everyone always wants to know, how do I make meatballs without eggs? It is really is simple to make egg free meatballs. Paleo meatballs are the perfect crowd pleaser. The entire family loves them and if I am trying to keep things healthy, I will simply eat mine with zoodles.

Meatballs are one of those things that have always felt like a lot of work, until now! All of the meatball recipes I made in the past contained eggs and breadcrumbs. When you are GF, breadcrumbs are harder to come by, somewhat pricey and just feel like a chore to make them yourself. Not only is this a super healthy meatball, but it is insanely easy to make. So, these Italian Whole 3o Meatballs are also Gluten Fee Meatballs Without Breadcrumbs.

If you want to keep this paleo serve with zoodles and your favorite paleo sauce. I served ours will gluten free noodles and French Bread from my cookbook. Everyone went crazy for them and there was plenty of leftovers the next day.

If you make the French Bread, it makes 2 loaves. Have one loaf with dinner and use the other loaf to make a meatball sub, yum!

These Whole 30 meatballs are also the perfect paleo meatball appetizer recipe for any gathering. It checks off all of the allergens since its just meat and veggies. These are perfect for everyone! You can dress them up fancy if you would like with some chopped basil or Italian parsley. Paleo Italian Meatballs are my favorite!

You can make these meatballs as big or as little as you want. If you want bite sized meatballs for appetizers you could get 35-40 from the recipe. We typically make ours very large and I get 20 or so of them.

Before experimenting with different ways to make them I would just fry them. I found that it dried them out and made them too crisp on the outside. I like a soft and juicy meatball. When you brown them in the pan it helps to keep the meatball in tact, then transferring it to a baking dish and baking them in the sauce allows the meatballs to soak up the moisture and flavor.

I had planned to freeze half of the meatballs, but they were so good that we finished them off the next day.

I grew up not eating homemade meatballs. The only ones I ever had (other than restaurants) were the frozen ones. My family is Spanish though and my grandma was the primary cook. I have always liked meatballs, but it wasn't something I got overly excited for...until now!

My husband always loved meatballs, and in fact I found out I was pregnant with our son shortly after craving meatballs (I was vegetarian at the time too). My kids love them and ask for them all of the time. That is another reason I created this recipe. I wanted a delicious, healthy, and simple meatball that I could turn to whenever they asked for them.

Paleo Meatballs no eggs

How do I throw these Paleo Meatballs that are also Egg Free together?

This recipe calls for 2 lbs. of ground meat. I used half ground turkey and half ground beef. This helped to make the recipe more affordable and a little leaner than using all beef.

You simply add all of your ingredients into a bowl and mix well.

Form them into meatballs and brown in a frying pan.

Pour some sauce onto the bottom of a baking dish, put the meatballs on top and pour more sauce on top.

Bake covered. Then uncover at the end.

You can also add some vegan mozzarella shreds on top if your feeling fancy.

This will be the perfect dinner to serve for guests, or just on a weeknight for your family. I haven't made them in the crock pot yet, but the next time I make these I would love to brown them on the stove top and then slow cook them in the crock pot. You could even brown them the night before and then pop them in the slow cooker in the morning before you head out to work.

They are even easy enough to get the kids involved. Here is little James after he made some.

I am confident this will become your go-to paleo meatball and egg free meatballs. Enjoy!

Prep Time 10 minutes

Cook Time 20 minutes

Total Time 30 minutes

Servings 20 Meatballs

Calories 135 kcal

Ingredients

2 lbs. Ground Beef you can also do half ground turkey and half ground beef

1 Onion diced

5 Cloves of Garlic diced

1 Bell Pepper diced

1 tsp. Oregano

117

1 tsp. Parsley

1 tsp. Basil

½ tsp. Sage

1 tsp. Garlic Powder

½ tsp. Rosemary

½ tsp. Marjoram

½ tsp. Thyme

¼ tsp. Pepper

1 tsp. Salt

4 Cups of your favorite spaghetti or marinara sauce.

Instructions

Preheat oven to 425°F.

Add all the ingredients except the sauce to a bowl and blend well with your hands.

Heat a large skillet on medium high heat.

Form and shape the meatballs with your hands.

Cook the meatballs in the skillet for 5 minutes.

Flip the meatballs and cook for another 5 minutes.

Pour 2 cups of spaghetti sauce on the bottom of the baking dish (9x13).

Transfer the meatballs to the baking dish and pour the remaining sauce on top of the meatballs.

Cover the dish with foil and bake for 20 minutes.

10. Remove from oven and serve. Enjoy!

Best Gluten Free Ready-Made Desserts

9th Annual Gluten-Free Awards:

1st Place Winner: SO Delicious Cashew Milk Snickerdoodle Frozen Dessert

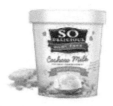

2nd Place Winner: Daiya New York Cheezecake

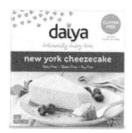

3rd Place Winner: Julie's Organic Gluten Free Ice Cream Sandwiches

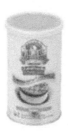

Other Great Products:

The Piping Gourmets Chocolate Mint Gluten-Free Whoopie Pies

Bubbies - Green Tea Mochi Ice Cream

Best Gluten Free Rolls

9th Annual Gluten-Free Awards:

1st Place Winner: Udi's Gluten Free Classic French Dinner Rolls

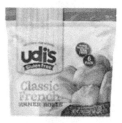

2nd Place Winner: Schär: Ciabatta Rolls

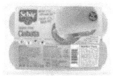

3rd Place Winner: Against the Grain - Rosemary Rolls

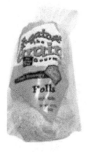

Other Great Products:

Schär: Sub Sandwich Rolls

Three Bakers' Whole Grain Hoagie Roll

Bread SRSLY Gluten-Free Sourdough Sandwich Rolls

Best Gluten Free Sauces

9th Annual Gluten-Free Awards:

1st Place Winner: Stubb's BBQ Sauce - Original

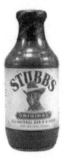

2nd Place Winner: San-J Organic Gluten Free Tamari Soy Sauce (Gold Label)

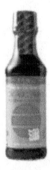

3rd Place Winner: OrganicVille BBQ Sauce Original

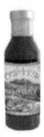

Other Great Products:

Saffron Road Lemongrass Basil Simmer Sauce

Claude's: Barbeque Brisket Marinade Sauce

Blue Top Brand Cilantro Serrano Creamy Hot Sauce

DID YOU KNOW?

CELIAC DISEASE CASES DOUBLE EVERY 15 YEARS IN THE UNITED STATES

Quoted from:
17th International Celiac Disease
Symposium in New Delhi, India

Best Gluten Free Snack Bars

9th Annual Gluten-Free Awards:

1st Place Winner: LÄRABAR Peanut Butter & Jelly

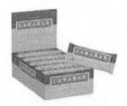

2nd Place Winner: Enjoy Life Foods | Chocolate Marshmallow Grain & Seed Bars

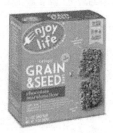

3rd Place Winner: The GFB Peanut Butter Bar

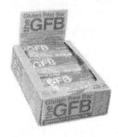

Other Great Products:

Bobo's® Coconut Oat Bar

ProBar Coconut Almond Bite Bar

thinkKIDS, Kids Protein Bar

Best Gluten Free Social Media Platforms

9th Annual Gluten-Free Awards:

1st Place Winner: Facebook

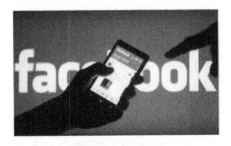

2nd Place Winner: Pinterest

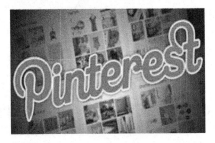

3rd Place Winner: Instagram

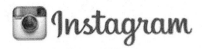

Other Great Social Media Platforms:

Google +

Twitter

Freedible

Meet-Up

Linked In

Best Gluten Free Soups

9th Annual Gluten-Free Awards:

1st Place Winner: Progresso Soup Rich & Hearty New England Clam Chowder Soup Gluten Free

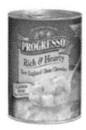

2nd Place Winner: Amy's Organic Thai Coconut Soup (Tom Kha Phak)

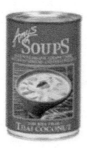

3rd Place Winner: Gluten Free Cafe Chicken Noodle Soup

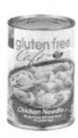

Other Great Products:

Boulder Organic Foods Roasted Tomato Basil Soup

Namaste Foods Gluten Free Chicken Noodle Soup

Dr McDougall's Gluten Free Rice Noodle Asian Soup, Sesame Chicken

San-J White Miso Soup Envelopes

Savory Choice Pho Chicken Broth Concentrate

Best Gluten Free Stuffing

9th Annual Gluten-Free Awards:

1st Place Winner: ADLI: liveGfree Gluten Free Chicken Stuffing

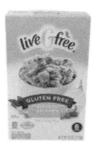

2nd Place Winner: Ian's Natural Foods Gluten Free Savory Stuffing

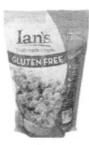

3rd Place Winner: Three Bakers' Herb Seasoned Stuffing Mix

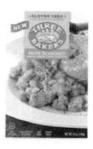

Other Great Products:

Aleia's Gluten Free Savory Stuffing

Williams Sonoma Gluten-Free Stuffing

Gordon Rhodes - Gluten Free Sage and Onion Stuffing Mix

100% Gluten-Free Eateries

Jackie Aanonsen McEwan, founder of Gluten Free Follow Me

Whether you have a gluten sensitivity, allergy, or celiac disease, you have to be incredibly careful when dining out. Thankfully, there are some eateries that represent themselves as 100% gluten-free and thus should be safe for those with celiac disease. If you have celiac disease and only feel comfortable eating out at a 100% gluten-free restaurant, that's understandable and completely up to you. I share my tips on how to dine out gluten-free here.

I personally review everything that's featured on glutenfreefollowme.com including all of the restaurants. Below is a list of all the 100% gluten-free eateries I've been to. There are 58 of them. California and New York have a ton, and there are also some in Pennsylvania, Colorado, Connecticut, Florida, Illinois, New Jersey, Oregon and Italy. How many have you been to?! And which ones am I missing?!

I've broken the eateries down by location. You can also customize your own restaurant searches for nearly 1,500 restaurants here. On the Restaurants page, you can filter by 100% gluten-free on the "Has To Be" filter to see all of the 100% gluten-free eateries. Please note that food offerings can change at any time so I urge you to ask the eatery before dining to make sure they are still 100% gluten-free. Enjoy!

100% Gluten-Free Eateries in New York:

Sit-Down Restaurants:

Senza Gluten (Greenwich Village) — Italian food

The Little Beet Table (Flatiron) — American food

Risotteria Melotti (East Village) — Italian food

Colors (NoHo) — American food

Cosme (Flatiron) — Mexican food

Grab & Go Eateries:

The Little Beet (Flatiron, Midtown West, Midtown East, The Pennsy above Penn Station, & Garden City) — veggie oriented

Hu Kitchen (Union Square & Upper East Side) — veggie oriented

Inday (Flatiron) — Indian food

Springbone Kitchen (Greenwich Village) — real food

Tap (Upper West Side) — Brazilian tapiocaria

Oca (NoHo) — Brazilian tapiocaria

Magic Mix Juicery (FiDi) — organic restaurant; 100% dairy free

Indie Fresh (Hell's Kitchen) — juice bar

Organic Pharmer (Rye Brook & Scarsdale) — plant-based; 100% dairy free

Bakeries:

Senza Gluten Cafe & Bakery (Greenwich Village) — cafe & bakery

Erin McKenna's Bakery (Lower East Side) — bakery; 100% vegan & dairy free

By The Way Bakery (Upper West Side, Upper East Side, Westchester) — bakery; 100% dairy free

NoGlu (Upper East Side) — bakery

Tu-Lu's Gluten Free Bakery (East Village) — bakery

100% Gluten-Free Eateries in California:

Sit-Down Restaurants:

Shojin (Culver City) — macrobiotic & vegan Japanese food

Grab & Go Eateries:

Beaming (Santa Monica, Brentwood, Century City, West Hollywood in LA; La Jolla; La Costa; Del Mar) — superfood cafe

Wild Living Foods (Downtown LA) — plant-based

Powerplant Superfood Café (Mid-City in LA) — superfood cafe

Peace Pies (San Diego) — 100% vegan, dairy free, & raw

Green Table (Santa Barbara) — organic restaurant

Sweetfin Poke (Santa Monica, Woodland Hills, Larchmont, Westwood, Beverly Grove, Downtown LA, Silverlake in LA; San Diego) — poke

Stuff'd (Hollywood in LA) — dumpling shop

Food Harmonics (Ojai) — organic cafe

Beefsteak (West Hollywood in LA) — plant-based

Lifehouse Tonics (West Hollywood in LA) — tonics & elixirs

Open Source Organics (West Hollywood in LA) — 100% vegan, dairy free, raw, & organic

Bakeries:

Lilac Patisserie (Santa Barbara) — bakery

Breakaway Bakery (Mid-City in LA) — bakery

Twice Baked Baking Company (Long Beach) — bakery

Erin McKenna's Bakery (Larchmont in LA) — bakery; 100% vegan & dairy free

Joy And Sweets (Culver City in LA) — bakery

The Good Cookies (Torrance) — bakery

Kirari West Bakery (Redondo Beach) — bakery

Mariposa Baking (San Francisco & Oakland) — bakery

Pomegranate (Beverly Grove in LA) — bakery; 100% vegan & dairy free

Rawberri (West Hollywood in LA) — ice cream & juice bar; 100% dairy free

Kippy's Ice Cream Shop (Venice in LA) — ice cream; 100% dairy free

Sensitive Sweets (Fountain Valley) — bakery; 100% vegan & nut free

100% Gluten-Free Eateries in Pennsylvania:

Eden Bistro (Pittsburgh) — cafe; 100% vegan

Sweet Freedom Bakery (Pittsburgh) — bakery; 100% vegan & dairy free

P.S. & Co (Philadelphia) — bakery & cafe; 100% vegan & dairy free

Gluuteny (Philadelphia) — bakery; 100% dairy free

100% Gluten-Free Eateries in Colorado:

Kim and Jake's Cakes (Boulder) — bakery

100% Gluten-Free Eateries in Connecticut:

By The Way Bakery (Greenwich) — bakery; 100% dairy free

100% Gluten-Free Eateries in Florida:

Erin McKenna's Bakery (Orlando) — bakery; 100% vegan & dairy free

100% Gluten-Free Eateries in Illinois:

Wheat's End Cafe (Chicago) — cafe & bakery

The Little Beet Table (Chicago) — American food

100% Gluten-Free Eateries in New Jersey:

OM Sweet Home (Hoboken) — bakery; 100% vegan & dairy free

Mo'pweeze Bakery (Denville) — bakery; 100% vegan & dairy free

100% Gluten-Free Eateries in Oregon:

Petunia's Pies & Pastries (Portland) — bakery; 100% vegan & dairy free

New Cascadia Traditional Bakery (Portland) — bakery

Ground Breaker Brewing (Portland) — brewery & gastropub

100% Gluten-Free Eateries in Italy:

Ristorante Quinoa (Florence) — Asian & Italian & Mediterranean food

Best Gluten Free Summer Camps

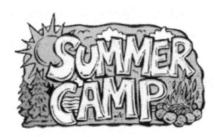

9th Annual Gluten-Free Awards:

1st Place Winner: Gluten-Free Fun CampMaple Lake, Minnesota

2nd Place Winner: Gluten-Free Overnight CampMiddleville, Michigan

3rd Place Winner: GIG (Gluten Intolerance Group) Kids Camp EastCamp KanataWake Forest, North Carolina

Other Great Camps:

The Great Gluten Escape at GilmontGilmer, Texas

Camp CeliacLivermore, California

GIG Kids Camp WestCamp SealthVashon Island, Washington

CDF Camp Gluten-Free Camp Fire Camp NawakwaSan Bernardino Mountains, CA

Camp WeekaneatitWarm Springs, Georgia

Gluten Detectives Camp (Day Camp)Bloomington, Minnesota

Camp CeliacNorth Scituate, Rhode Island

Timber Lake CampShandaken, New York

International Sports Training CampPocono Mountains,Pennsylvania

Camp EmersonHinsdale, Massachusetts

Appel Farm Arts CampElmer, New Jersey

Camp TAG - Williamstown, New Jersey

Camp Eagle HillElizaville, New York

Emma Kaufmann CampMorgantown, West Virginia

Foundation for Children & Youth with Diabetes Camp UTADAWest Jordan, Utah

Camp Silly-YakBrigadoon VillageAylesford, Nova Scotia

Camp TAG Lebanon, Ohio at YMCA's Camp Kern.

FAACT's Annual Teen Retreat

Clear Creek CampGreen's Canyon, Utah (Serves Alpine School District children)

Positive Quotes from Kids with Celiac

Jessica Hanson, Founder of Tasty Meditation

www.TastyMeditation.com

Throughout the years I've chatted with several children who have Celiac Disease. Each one was bright, well spoken, and empathetic, and they inspired me to create this post. I recently sent out messages on the Facebook and twitter-verse asking parents to chat with their kids about the positive side of Celiac Disease and send me what their kids had to say (thanks to everyone who participated!). These kids are the BEST. While I'm stressing about food to eat at a wedding, these kids are conquering the universe! I hope this post will be inspiring to both children and adults. It's certainly been inspiring to me.

What is the best part about having Celiac Disease?

"You get to see your insides on pictures after the biopsy"

"You feel amazing!" (10 years old, diagnosed 1 month ago)

"The best part is you are aware and can fix the problem so you feel better."

"I don't have to be sick" (9 years old, diagnosed at age 3)

"My mum makes me so many different foods I don't feel I am missing out."

"At class parties everyone else gets store bought cupcakes, but I get homemade cupcakes that are way better."

"I get bigger treats" (4 years old, diagnosed 8 months ago)

"The gluten free pizza tastes better than the pizza with gluten." (6 years old, diagnosed 1 week ago)

"You don't have to share your yummy food as most think gluten free food is not good and has no taste."

"If there is a food that I really don't want to eat at a party, I can just say – hmmm, I'm not sure if that is gluten free. Sorry I can't eat it!"

"I don't eat a lot of junk food and other foods that I know I shouldn't eat that much." (9 years old)

"I am a kid that likes to eat" (7 years old, diagnosed at age 3)

"Sometimes I get bigger treats than the other kids" (7 years old, diagnosed at 18 months)

"I feel special because mum makes everything at home for me, and my brother and dad have to eat the same food! hahaha"

"That I'm like my mom" (8 years old, diagnosed at age 3)

"I love going to the Allergy Show in London with my mom every year. I like trying all the different foods – especially pizza! – and also meeting up with my mom's Twitter friends. Also I love eating out at safe restaurants." (11 years old, diagnosed age 5)

"The best part of having Coeliac Disease as a 17 year old is that I don't have to share my food! I also love sharing my food finds on Instagram and in Facebook support groups. There's a community that I would never have been involved in without having Coeliac Disease."

"You are not like everybody else. We are different."

What is better now that you eat gluten free?

"I don't feel sick anymore" (9 years old, diagnosed at age 3)

"Much less pain! More people are beginning to understand what it's like for me. The ready made food is always improving too."

"I don't really remember eating gluten containing foods. I'm learning new cooking and baking skills which I love!" (11 years old, diagnosed age 5)

"You don't throw up."

"Everything because I feel better and I can eat cake!"

"I always get to take my own food and I always know I will have food I like for lunch in school."

"I'm not sick anymore! I prefer natural gluten free foods to begin with, like fruits and vegetables" (9 years old)

"I'm not throwing up anymore and it's better for my body." (6 years old, diagnosed 1 week ago)

"More cheese!" (his parents are vegan) (10 years old, diagnosed 1 month ago)

"That I don't get sick" (7 years old, diagnosed at age 3)

"My health. I feel better all around" (4 years old, diagnosed 8 months ago)

"I don't have any more tummy aches" (8 years old, diagnosed at age 3)

"I'm not so sad" (7 years old, diagnosed at 18 months)

"I make healthier choices because I guess I don't have a choice. It forces me to eat better because I can't eat the pizza and junk food that kids eat at birthday parties."

"Now I eat gluten free I don't feel ill at all, I have energy again, and I don't feel sick constantly. I also know I'm not making my insides unhappy!"

What would you want to tell other kids your age who just got diagnosed?

"You are not alone. Don't need to feel different." (4 years old, diagnosed 8 months ago)

"It's nothing but food so it's no big deal."

"You can make almost anything without gluten."

"It's a-ok and you can eat lots of things even cake and sometimes it's even better than regular cake. Can you tell I like cake?"

"It's okay, you just have to get used to eating gluten free. There's a lot of great gluten free foods out there. I don't feel like I miss anything." (9 years old)

"It gets better! I cried at first but it's really not bad."

"That gluten free foods are good" (7 years old, diagnosed at age 3)

"It feels easier the longer you have it" (8 years old, diagnosed at age 3)

"You're not the only one and there are other Celiac kids" (7 years old, diagnosed at 18 months)

"If someone is teasing you about the food like 'You can't eat gluten' you can say 'hey stop it!' If they don't stop you can tell their parents." (6 years old, diagnosed 1 week ago)

"Don't be scared, the food isn't as bad as everyone thinks and in some cases it's easy for your mum to make your favorite food gluten free."

"Our cupcakes are way better than grocery store cake."

"Don't be worried. You'll miss the foods you used to eat, but it will get easier. Always read labels and ask lots of questions when you eat out." (11 years old, diagnosed age 5)

"As a 17-year-old, you think it's awful but honestly it's not bad at all! There are groups that have events and provide support. Socially, your friends will understand and accommodate you, but you have to stick to your guns and be gluten free because it's what your body needs!"

"It's not as hard after you get used to it" (9 years old, diagnosed at age 3)

"Class parties where everyone is eating cake except for you may suck at first, but in a year or so you'll realize that it's not a big deal at all. I don't care now. I can eat a cupcake anytime."

"The most important thing is to understand about Celiac and understanding everything you can and can't eat so then you can educate others when they ask you questions."

"It'll be o.k." (10 years old, diagnosed 1 month ago)

Best Gluten Free Supplements

9th Annual Gluten-Free Awards:

1st Place Winner: Nature's Bounty Daily Multi

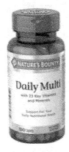

2nd Place Winner: Vega

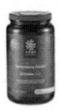

3rd Place Winner: Olly

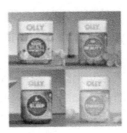

Other Great Products:

MegaFood – Daily

Jarrow - Organic Plant Protein Salted Caramel

Plant Fusion Protein

Standard Process Whole Food Fiber

Silver Fern Ultimate Probiotic

Growing Naturals Rice Protein

Best Gluten Free Tortilla or Wrap

9th Annual Gluten-Free Awards:

1st Place Winner: Mission Soft Taco Gluten Free 8ct

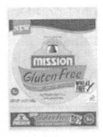

2nd Place Winner: ALDI: liveGfree Spinach Wraps

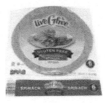

3rd Place Winner: Guerrero Corn Tortillas

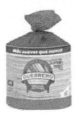

Other Great Products:

BFree Multigrain Wrap

La Banderita Corn Tortillas

Siete Almond Flour Tortillas

Raw Wraps Spinach- Gluten & Soy Free, Vegan & Raw, Paleo (Quinoa Seeds)

DID YOU KNOW?

CELIAC DISEASE IS NOW AT THE CENTER-STAGE OF THE SCIENTIFIC WORLD. THE PAST DECADE HAS BEEN VERY EXCITING AND PRODUCTIVE IN TERMS OF DIAGNOSTICS AND UNDERSTANDING THE BIOLOGY OF CELIAC DISEASE. WHILE GLUTEN-FREE DIET IS THE BEST MODE OF TREATMENT, MANY OTHER TARGETS FOR CONTROL OF THE IMMUNE-PATHOGENESIS OF CELIAC DISEASE ARE NOW ACTIVELY EXPLORED, SOME OF THEM HAVE REACHED EVEN PHASE 2 AND PHASE 3 CLINICAL TRIALS.

Quoted from:
17th International Celiac Disease
Symposium in New Delhi, India

Best Gluten Free Vacation Destinations

9th Annual Gluten-Free Awards:

1st Place Winner: Walt Disney World

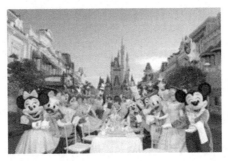

2nd Place Winner: Italy

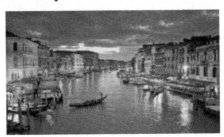

3rd Place Winner: New York City

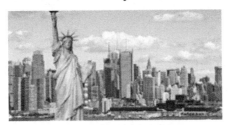

Other Great Vacation Locations:

Royal Caribbean Cruises

Disney Cruises

London, England

Reykjavik - Capital of Iceland

GIG Generation Gluten Free Teen Summit

10 Tips for Gluten Free Air Travel

Diana Duangnet, Creator at travelfarglutenfree.com

Air travel can be stressful and having to eat gluten free can add even more undue stress. Follow these 10 tips before heading to the airport to help ease your mind and feed your hungry tummy during your travels.

1. Book a meal in advance

For international flights with food service, you can book a special gluten free meal in advance. Many times, you can do it at the time of booking, if not right after the booking. Make sure to put in special meal requests at least 24 to 48 hours before the flight.

2 Gluten free bars

Pack gluten free protein bars and granola bars to snack on during the fight and for when you arrive at your destination. Always bring bars in your purse or pocket when you're out and about. You never know if you'll be out longer than expected and not be able to find gluten free food nearby when hunger strikes.

3. Travel friendly food

Make sure to pack travel friendly food. Food that can easily pass through security and travels well without refrigeration include:

Fresh fruit: grapes, bananas, apples, pears

Dried fruit: mango slices, banana chips

Beef jerky

Rice cakes and crackers

Nuts and trail mix

Gluten free muffins

Corn or potato chips

Tuna packets, single serving

4. Instant oatmeal

Pack single serving instant oatmeal packets for a quick, hot meal. You can request hot water from coffee shops in the airport or from the flight attendants on board the plane.

5. Sandwich or wrap

Make and pack gluten free sandwiches or wraps. It's an easy to make meal when you want something heartier than a snack or protein bar.

6. Zip Lock It

Don't use aluminum foil to wrap your food, it interferes with the x-ray machine. Pack your nuts, crackers, muffins, sandwiches, and/or wraps in plastic zip lock bags. It'll also be easier for TSA to look at your food items when they pull you aside, which they will with an abundant of food.

7. Freeze "liquid" and "gel" items

I got this tip from TSA themselves as they were throwing away my egg salad and salsa. If it's frozen it won't be considered a liquid or gel and will pass through security.

8. Pack all your food in one bag

Make it easy for TSA, and yourself, and pack all your food items in one bag. I usually use a small or medium sized reusable grocery bag for all my food items. If they flag you for your food, which they will if you have a lot, it'll be easy for them to examine the food you have.

9. Get a doctor's note

To avoid getting your food items tossed by TSA, ask your doctor to write you a note to state that it is medically necessary for you to have your own packed food.

10. Airport food

You'll be surprised at the number of chain and fast food restaurants that have gluten free options, including Chick-fil-a, Chili's, PF Chang's, and Five Guys. If you're unsure of what to eat, stick to naturally gluten free foods, including grilled chicken, steam vegetables, and fruits.

Best Gluten Free Website

9th Annual Gluten-Free Awards:

1st Place Winner: gfJules.com

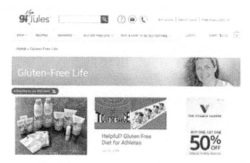

2nd Place Winner: Gluten Free Watch Dog

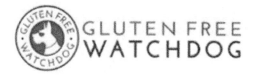

3rd Place Winner: Celiac and the Beast

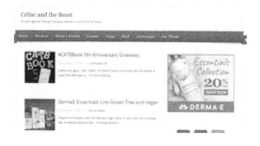

Other Great Gluten Free Websites:

Cure Celiac Disease.org

Gluten Free Travel Site

Gluten Free Globetrotter

Travel Far Gluten Free

GlutenfreeGlobalicious

HaleLife Online Expo

Grain Changer

Strength and Sunshine

BuenQamino

DID YOU KNOW?

AFTER BEING WELL RECOGNIZED IN EUROPE AND AMERICA, CELIAC DISEASE IS NOW GETTING RECOGNIZED IN ASIAN COUNTRIES. IT IS PREDICTED THAT THE NUMBER OF PATIENTS WITH CELIAC DISEASE IN ASIA MAY SURPASS THE NUMBERS PRESENT IN REST OF THE WORLD.

Quoted from:
17th International Celiac Disease Symposium in New Delhi, India

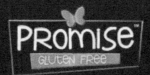

Baked In-Store Range

Innovative new range of baked in-store gluten free sourdough loaves that bake in the bag to produce crusty, fresh gluten free bread for the first time ever.

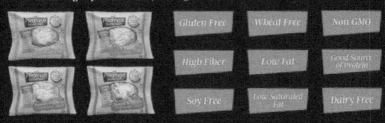

Product Description	Weight	Units Per Case	Unit UPC	Case UPC	Shelf Life	
					Thawed	Frozen
Promise Gluten Free Rustic White Sourdough ISB Loaf	14.1oz	3	813002020507	05391520163500	5 Days	365 Days
Promise Gluten Free 7 Seed Sourdough ISB Loaf	14.1oz	3	813002020491	05391520163517	5 Days	365 Days
Promise Gluten Free Seeded Rosemary & Olive Oil Sourdough ISB Loaf	14.1oz	3	813002020552	05391520163535	5 Days	365 Days
Promise Gluten Free Seeds & Fruits Sourdough ISB Loaf	14.1oz	3	813002020545	05391520163548	5 Days	365 Days

Suitable for Vegetarians

Gluten Free Product Registration

By submitting your products into The Gluten Free Awards (GFA), you are automatically entering products into the Annual Gluten Free Buyers Guide. There are only 10 slots available in each category and we limit brands to 3 submissions per category. If you are a marketer representing multiple brands, this typically will not apply. Slots can fill quickly so we recommend submitting your registration ASAP. The absolute deadline for registration is August 22nd however, we cannot guarantee you that the category is already full.

"How do I get into the Gluten Free Awards?"

How it works:

1. Fill out the registration form by adding the quantities and product names.

(A free half page ad is given for every 5 products or full-page ad for 10 products.)

2. If wanted, add additional ad space to registration.

3. Email the registration form to Jayme@GlutenFreeBuyersGuide.com

4. We will follow up with a confirmation and invoice.

If you have any questions call customer support at 828-446-1952

"Wait, I have tons of questions still"

Most common questions:

Q: I am having a hard time understanding how to submit or products.

A: Using this Registration Form will help. If lost, don't hesitate to call or email. 828-455-9734

Q: What are the image specs you need?

A: Our graphic team just needs images that are PDF, JPEG or PNG at 300 dpi or greater. The team will normally resize images based on the publishing media. Normally the product pictures and descriptions from your website will work just fine.

Q: Is there a word count for product descriptions?

A: No, we normally don't use product descriptions just product names and images.

Q: If we submit 10 products do we get 1 free full-page ad and 2 free half page ads?

A: Sorry, please choose one or the other. You can always purchase additional ad space.

Q: Can we run a full-page ad without entering the awards program?

A: Yes.

Q: Do we need to send you product samples?

A: No. The gluten-free community votes for your products.

Q: Will we be in the guide if we don't win an award?

A: Yes, all products submitted will be visible as nominees.

Q: Can we use the GFA Nominee and Winner Badge on our product packaging, website and other related media?

A: Yes, we highly recommend using the badges to differentiate your products from the rest. If you happen to need higher resolution images don't hesitate to ask. Read our media terms here.

Need to talk about your order or have questions? Give us a call.

828-455-9734

or email

Josh@GlutenFreeBuyersGuide.com

From our family to yours have a happy and healthy gluten free lifestyle.

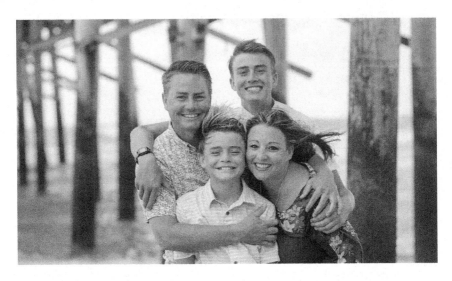

The Schieffer Family

Josh (Dad with Celiac) Chief Marketing Officer

Jayme (Mom) VP Operations

Blake (18)

Jacob (14 Celiac)

Keep up to date with us, the awards, and future buyer guides at
GlutenFreeBuyersGuide.com

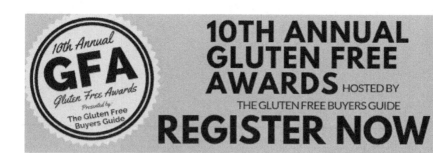

Made in the USA
Columbia, SC
19 September 2019